Sirtfood Diet For Beginners

Complete Beginners Guide To The Sirtfood Diet

(With Delicious Recipes And Meal Plan)

Helen Amato

Introduction

I want to thank you and congratulate you for purchasing the book, *"Sirtfood Diet for Beginners."*

Have you been trying to lose weight for a while?

Are you on the verge of giving up losing weight because nothing seems to work?

Would you like to know an effective way to lose weight and take steps to actually encourage your body to lose weight?

If the above scenarios describe you then this book is what you need because in it you will learn about the sirtfood diet that has been shown to be quite effective for weight loss. A number of celebrities have followed the diet with great results and you too can try it, what have you got to lose anyway.

To help you transition into the diet successfully, this book will help you understand what the diet entails, the foods to eat while on the diet, amazing benefits of adopting the diet other than weight loss, tasty recipes to try out and a meal plan to get you started.

I hope you enjoy it!

PS: I'd like your feedback. If you are happy with this book, please leave a review on Amazon.

Please leave a review for this book on Amazon by visiting the page below:

https://amzn.to/2VMR5qr

PSS: The ebook version has color images so be sure to check that out.

Table of Contents

Basics Of The Sirtfood Diet

Sirtfood diet is a diet that focuses on eating foods that are high in "sirtuin activators." The term **sirtuins** refers to a group of 7 proteins that protect and regulate various bodily functions. In addition to protecting our bodies from inflammation and premature death, research shows that the 7 sirtuins (SIRT 1-7) are also effective in boosting muscle growth, regulating metabolism, and promoting weight loss. Additional studies show that Sirtuin 1, for instance, helps control insulin secretion, regulate glucose tolerance, and regulates lipid mobilization from cells.

From these scientifically proven benefits, the sirtfood diet can promote rapid weight loss without muscle protein breakdown, while still protecting you from chronic diseases altogether. However, to achieve all this, you also need to incorporate a bit of calorie restriction along with eating sirtuin-promoting foods.

So, where did this diet come from? Two health consultants and authors, Glen Matten and Aidan Goggins invented the diet. In their book entitled "the Sirtfood Diet," the duo suggest a meal plan that includes drinking three sirtfood green juices for a few days in the diet along with a balanced diet comprising of sirtfood-rich meals.

Let us now break down the diet to understand it better:

The Sirtfood diet is comprised of two phases that last a total of 21 days. After the 3 weeks, you are free to eat without calorie restriction as long as you focus on sirtfood-rich meals, which means that you aren't restricted to eating only the sirtuins activators, but you can also add other ingredients. Also, since the signature of the Sirtfood diet is green juice, you'll need to make enough amounts for 3 times per day serving. Here is what you'll need to do in the two phases of the diet:

Phase One

This phase lasts for a total of 7 days, and it's the strictest in terms of calorie restriction! The phase's goal is to help you kick start your weight loss program and, if well followed, can help you shed at least 3.2 kg (7 pounds) in a week.

In the first three days of the week, you'll need to limit calorie intake to 1000 while drinking three green juices in a day, along with one sirtfood meal. An ideal meal could be anything from buckwheat noodles to sirtfood omelet or miso-glazed tofu. In the next four days within the week of the diet, you can increase your calorie intake to 1,500 by taking in 2 green juices in a day along with two main meals from the Sirtfood diet.

Phase Two

The second phase, also referred to as the "maintenance phase," goes for 14 days, and its role is to help you constantly lose weight without the need for calorie restriction. Here you should drink just one green juice a day along with 3 "balanced" meals rich in Sirt foods.

After The 3 Weeks

You should continue incorporating sirtfoods in your diet regularly, even after completing the two phases along with one serving of green juice a day. However, in some circumstances, you may need to repeat any of the two phases to jump-start a weight-loss plateau. For better results, you should make the Sirtfood diet more of a lifestyle change as opposed to a one-term quick-weight-loss diet.

So which foods should you include in your green juice and other regular meals? Here are the top foods rich in sirtuins, also the "top 20 sirtfoods":

Sirtfood Diet Food List

We will start by looking at the top sirtfoods, which include:

- Coffee

- Capers

- Blueberries

- Red chicory

- Bird's eye chili

- Arugula (rocket)

- Walnuts

- Turmeric

- Buckwheat

- Matcha green tea

- Dark chocolate (with 85% cocoa)

- Extra virgin olive oil

- Parsley

- Soy

- Onions

- Strawberries

- Red wine

- Kale

- Medjool dates

- Lovage or celery leaves

Note

While many people are only conversant with the top 20 sirtfoods, there are, however, **hundreds of foods** that also have a significant concentration of sirtuin proteins. Therefore you have a variety of foods to choose from as far as sirtuin-activating nutrients are concerned, ranging from veggies such as broccoli, whole grains, meat, and fruits, among others.

Here are the comprehensive sirtfood food groups along with sirtuin trigger foods:

Other Sirtfoods And "Sirtuin Activators"

1. Resveratrol

Various studies have proven that indeed **resveratrol** is a sirtuin activator in that it mimics calorie restriction by stimulating the Sirtuin 1 (SIRT1). This SIRT 1 activator indirectly helps trigger the activation of SIRT1 genes, which ultimately boost sirtuin-1 levels in the body cells. Research has shown that resveratrol-induced increase in sirtuin-1 stimulates various parameters linked to the regulation of cellular aging. Resveratrol, along with calorie restriction, results in an increased SIRT gene expression, which brings benefits such as the breakdown of body lipids.

Here are foods that are high in sirtuin-activating resveratrol:

Berries:

Mulberries, Lingo berries, Cranberries, Bilberries, Blueberries, Strawberries

Nuts

Pistachios

Other fruits

Red currants, Jackfruit skin, Fresh grapes

Others

Milk chocolate, Dark chocolate, Cocoa powder, Peanut butter, Peanuts, Red grape juice, Red wine

2. Polyphenols

These are antioxidant-rich compounds found in bitter veggies and other foods whose main role is giving plants their color (anthocyanins) and defending them from attack. Generally, foods that make your mouth pucker often contain polyphenols such as red wine, chili, or strongly brewed tea.

Research has shown that polyphenols-rich foods not only help facilitate weight loss, improve digestion, control diabetes, and fight cardiovascular diseases but also help modulate sirtuins. Here are foods rich in sirtuin activator polyphenols:

- Green tea, black tea, red wine, cocoa, and coffee

- Green olives, black olives, and extra-virgin olive oil

- Spices such as ginger, chili, paprika, cinnamon, curry powder, cumin, capers, cloves

- Dark chocolate

- Herbs such as sage, oregano, rosemary, parsley, basil, thyme, marjoram, and lemon verbena

- Dark berries such as blackberries, raspberry, strawberry, blueberry, and black elderberry

- Nuts and seeds such as walnuts, almonds, pecans, hazelnuts, chestnuts, celery seeds and flax seeds

- Veggies such as broccoli, spinach, red onion, green chicory, artichokes, curly endive and sweet potato

- Fruits and juices such as apricot, lemon juice, blood orange juice, peach, pomegranate juice and apple juice

3. Melatonin

Foods high in melatonin are also considered sirtuin activators, among them the tryptophan-rich foods such as seafood, poultry, and dairy. Such foods include:

- Fruits such as grapes, bananas, tomatoes, olives, cherries, and pomegranate

- Veggies such as cucumber, broccoli, asparagus, corn

- Grains among them rolled oats, barley, and rice

- Nuts and seeds such as flax seeds, sunflower seeds, and walnuts

4. DHA (Docosahexaenoic Acid)

DHA has been proven to increase the concentration of Sirtuin 1 in body cells and help boost the vascular function of cerebral flow and blood vessels. This omega-3 fatty acid can thereby help boost blood flow, metabolism, and other bodily processes such as fat breakdown. DHA is mainly found in fish and seafood but may also be made in the body from the alpha-linolenic acids (ALAs), which are found in plants.

Here is a list of food rich in the sirtuin 1 activator DHA:

- Snow Crab (Queen Crab)

- Clams

- Pickled Herring

- Fish Roe (Ikura, Caviar)

- Atlantic Cod

- Oysters

- Mussels

- Trout

- Tuna

- Fish (Salmon)

5. Zinc

Studies show that zinc is vital in maintaining the optimal activity of the sirtuin 1 protein. Zinc is also important for the synthesis of DNA, triggering various body enzymes, building proteins, and boosting the immune system. While zinc is mostly found in meat, fish, and other seafood, it's also found in plants too. Here the sources of SIRT 1 booster zinc:

- Lean Pork Chops

- Chicken Leg

- Beef (Chuck Steak)

- Oysters

- Salmon

- Mushrooms

- Oatmeal

- Low-Fat Yogurt

- Lentils

- Hemp Seeds

- Firm Tofu

From the above information, no doubt there are hundreds of sirtuin-activating super-foods that you can eat. Let us now take an in-depth look at how sirtfoods facilitate weight loss.

Benefits Of The Sirtfood Diet

Let us now learn how you stand to benefit by adopting the sirtfood diet:

Weight Loss

A pilot study that comprised of 39 people clearly showed how effective this diet is for weight loss. In the study, the participants who followed the diet for one week and exercised daily lost an average of 7 pounds in 7 days! Better still, the participants maintained muscle mass with some gaining extra muscle mass though the study didn't follow up their progress beyond the one week of Sirtfood dieting.

Also, since the diet encourages calorie restriction in addition to eating sirtfoods, you will lose weight. When you deprive your body of energy, it eventually starts utilizing all its **emergency stores**, which is the glycogen (stored glucose), body fat, and the muscle.

According to studies, within seven days of extreme calorie restriction, you'll lose significant body weight with a third of the weight loss coming from "body fat" and the other two-thirds coming from glycogen, water, and muscle. To put this into perspective, each glycogen molecule needs 3 to 4 molecules of water to be stored in body tissues for future use. Thus utilization of glycogen into energy directly leads to loss of the water in what is referred to as "water weight."

Helps Fight Chronic Diseases

Studies show that Sirtuin 1 and 2 help in the control of diabetes and obesity, while sirtuin 3 has antioxidant powers that help shield your body from oxidative stress. SIRT 4 helps suppress tumors and controls cellular metabolic response to DNA damage and helps reduce insulin secretion.

Also, sirtfoods such as turmeric possess inflammatory power that helps prevent you from chronic inflammation and related diseases. Furthermore, drinking green tea, a sirtfood, has been linked to a reduced risk of diabetes, stroke and can help lower blood pressure.

Increases lifespan

Research in animals such as mice shows that increased levels of sirtuin proteins can lead to a longer lifespan. In addition, during calorie restriction, sirtuins help trigger the body to burn fat for energy and boosts insulin sensitivity. A particular study found out that higher level of sirtuins leads to fat burn. Additional studies show that sirtuins have also been found to slow down the development of Alzheimer's and the growth of tumors.

While studies in mice have shown positive results in increasing lifespan, for now, no studies back up such effects of increased sirtuins in human. But there are efforts to make compounds that help boost sirtuins in human bodies and this will be the framework of studying effects of sirtuins in human.

While sirtfoods are rich in antioxidants and posses excellent anti-inflammatory properties, there are concerns that **extreme calorie restriction** with **1 sirtfood meal** and green juices may fail to address all your body's nutritional need.

Let us look at some challenges of adopting this diet:

Is The Sirtfood Diet Healthy And Sustainable?

While the intake of green juices and sirtfood foods can provide you with a variety of nutrients, minerals, and vitamins, some challenges come with the diet.

It can be highly restrictive

The Sirtfood diet recommends that you restrict calorie intake to 1000 and 1500 per day, which is extremely low for many people. To ensure that you don't feel hungry, drink lots of water, and focus on eating more vegetables, as they are filling and will enable you to maintain the low-calorie intake.

Low In Fiber

The first phase of the Sirtfood diet involves drinking green juices, which are low in fiber, a nutrient that you need to help you feel full. There are health concerns that juicing reduces the amount of fiber content you'd get from whole vegetables or fruits. To ensure you get your required fiber intake, make sure that the one sirtfood meal you have in phase one is high in fiber.

Can damage your relationship with food

If you don't have a healthy relationship with food, this diet is not for you. Limiting your food intake may cause your body to interpret the lack of sustenance as starvation or some kind of an attack. Therefore, you may tend to feel hungry most of the time. Ensure that you snack on low-calorie vegetables that will ensure you stick within the recommended calories.

Not everyone can try the Sirtfood diet

Since this diet is low in calorie intake, it is not advisable to try out the diet if you have diabetes or if you are living a very active lifestyle.

Let us now look at some recipes to try out:

Sirtfood Recipes

Breakfast Recipes

Breakfast Scramble

Serves 1

Ingredients

2 eggs

5g parsley, finely chopped

A handful of button mushrooms, thinly sliced

1 teaspoon extra virgin olive oil

20g kale, roughly chopped

1 teaspoon mild curry powder

1 teaspoon ground turmeric

Directions

1. Mix the curry powder and turmeric along with some water until you get a light paste.

2. Steam the kale in boiling water for approximately 2 to 3 minutes.

3. In a frying pan over medium heat, heat olive oil, and then fry the mushrooms until they begin to brown and soften, or for about 2 to 3 minutes.

4. Add in the eggs and spices and cook the mixture over medium heat.

5. Add in the kale and cook over medium heat for around 1 minute.

6. Add in the parsley, stir, switch off the heat, serve, and enjoy. You can top with a seed mixture and preferred saucer if you like.

Overnight Oats

Serves 2

Ingredients

For the oats

1 teaspoon honey

2 pinches of ground cinnamon

1 teaspoon matcha powder

375ml almond milk, rice or oat milk

2 teaspoon chia seeds

80g (3oz) rolled oats

For the topping:

A handful of mixed nuts

1 teaspoon pumpkin seeds

1 apple, peeled, cored and chopped

Directions

1. Make the oats earlier, preferably the previous night. Put the oats along with the chia seeds in a container or bowl.

2. In a separate jug or bowl, add in a tablespoon of almond milk to the matcha tea powder and use a hand-held whisk to whisk the mixture into a smooth paste.

3. Top the smooth paste with the remaining milk and blend the mixture well.

4. Pour the matcha and almond milk mixture over the prepared oats and then stir in honey and cinnamon.

5. Cover and pop the mixture into the refrigerator and keep it overnight.

6. Once ready to serve, serve the oats and top with chopped pumpkin, apple, nuts, and seeds.

Tasty Porridge

Serves 1

Ingredients

50g strawberries, hulled

1 teaspoon walnut butter or 4 chopped walnut halves

35g buckwheat flakes

1 Medjool date, chopped

200 ml dairy-free milk

Directions

1. Put the milk and the dates in a pan.

2. Heat the mixture gently and then add in the buckwheat flakes.

3. Cook until the porridge achieves your desired consistency.

4. Stir in the walnuts or walnut butter and top the porridge with the strawberries. Enjoy!

Smoked Salmon Omelet

Serves 1

Ingredients

1 teaspoon extra virgin olive oil

1 teaspoon parsley, chopped

10g rocket, chopped

1/2 teaspoon capers

100g smoked salmon, sliced

2 medium eggs

Directions

1. Crack the eggs into a medium bowl and then whisk.

2. Add in the parsley, rocket, capers, and the salmon.

3. In a nonstick frying pan, add some olive oil and heat until hot.

4. Add in the egg and salmon mixture and move this around the pan using a fish slice or a spatula until it's even.

5. Lower the heat and allow the omelet to cook until ready.

6. Slide a spatula around the edges of the omelet and fold it in half or roll it up. Enjoy.

Fried Eggs

Serves 4

Ingredients

2 ounces coconut oil

8 eggs

Salt and pepper

Directions

1. Add coconut oil to a pan and heat the oil over medium heat.

2. In a measuring cup or frying pan, crack all the 8 eggs then gently pour them into the pan.

3. To get eggs with the sunny side up, let the eggs cook on one side, and then cover the pan to help the eggs cook at the top.

4. Season with salt and pepper and then serve.

Breakfast Sausage Patties

Yields 12 Patties

Ingredients

1/2 teaspoon nutmeg

1/2 teaspoon cayenne pepper

1 teaspoon black pepper

1 teaspoon paprika

1 teaspoon thyme

1 teaspoon sage

1 teaspoon Celtic sea salt

1 lb. ground pork

Directions

1. Prepare a spice mix and then season the ground pork with it. Simply rub the spices on the meat using your hands.

2. Roll the spiced pork into 12 equal-sized patties and then pan fry them in a skillet until they are no longer pink in the

middle. This should require cooking 3 to 4 minutes per side over medium-high heat.

4. Serve and enjoy.

Breakfast Casserole

Serves 6

Ingredients

1/8 teaspoon pepper

1/4 teaspoon sea salt

1/2 cup almond or coconut milk

12 eggs

12 ounces broccoli chopped

2 cloves garlic minced

1 pound sausage or other ground meat, nitrate-free

1 tablespoon olive oil

1/2 teaspoon dry minced onion flakes, optional

Cheese for serving

Directions

1.Begin by cooking the garlic, sausage, and onion flakes if using over medium-high heat until the sausage or other ground meat is browned.

2.Add in broccoli and mix. Pour this mixture into a casserole dish.

3. Whisk together coconut or almond milk and eggs in a medium bowl, and add in pepper and salt.

4. Pour the mixture over the browned sausage and bake until the eggs are set and the top begins to brown; this should take 30 to 35 minutes.

Easy Omelet

Serves 1

Ingredients

1/2 cup mixed vegetables

1 tablespoon unsalted butter

2 tablespoons water

2 eggs

Directions

1. Begin by beating the eggs and the water until well incorporated.

2. In a frying pan, heat some butter until it's hot to the extent that it sizzles when you drop some water.

3. Pour in the egg and water mixture and then gradually push the cooked edges to the center to allow the uncooked parts to touch the hot surface. You should move and tilt the cooking pan when needed.

4. Cook the mixture until the egg is fully set and doesn't flow.

5. Fill the omelet with veggies.

6. Place the filling on the side of the omelet and fold the omelet in half using a pancake turner.

7. Transfer the omelet onto a plate, with the bottom side of the omelet facing up.

Breakfast Salad

Serves 4

Ingredients

For the Dressing:

1/2 teaspoon mixed herbs: dill, chervil or tarragon

1/4 teaspoon pepper

1/2 teaspoon salt

1 lemon, juiced

1 tablespoon Dijon mustard

1/4 cup olive oil

For the Salad

1 shallot, finely sliced, sautéed until crisp in oil

1 avocado, sliced

2 large eggs, soft or hard-boiled and peeled

1 teaspoon olive oil

1 small bunch asparagus, cooked

5 ounces arugula, washed and dried

Directions

1. To make the salad dressing, put all the ingredients in a small jar that has a tight-fitting lid. Shake the mixture until the contents have emulsified.

2. To make the salad, simply toss the dressing, asparagus, and the salad greens together.

3. Serve the salad and top with the sliced avocado. Garnish the breakfast salad with crispy shallots.

Veggie Omelet

Serves 2

Ingredients

5 egg whites

1 large egg

1-ounce mozzarella cheese

2 cups spinach, organic baby

4 onions, raw, medium, sliced

Directions

1. Preheat a pan or skillet.

2. Combine 5 egg whites with 1 egg, stir to mix, and then pour into a pan.

3. Cook the eggs until set on one side.

4. Flip over the egg; add the onions, cheese, and spinach on the top, and then fold. Serve and enjoy!

Sirtfood Muesli

Serves 1

Ingredients

100g strawberries, hulled and chopped

100g plain yogurt

10g cocoa nibs

15g walnuts, chopped

40g Medjool dates, pitted and chopped

15g coconut flakes or desiccated coconut

10g buckwheat puffs

20g buckwheat flakes

Directions

1. Combine all the ingredients apart from the yogurt and strawberries unless if you're serving the muesli right away.

2. In case you want to make the muesli the night before or in bulk, just mix the dry ingredients and keep them in a well-sealed container.

3. The following day you can just add in the yogurt and strawberries and then serve.

Lunch Recipes

Chicken with Kale and Salsa

Serves 1

Ingredients

50g buckwheat

1 teaspoon chopped fresh ginger

20g red onion, sliced

50g kale, chopped

1 tablespoon extra virgin olive oil

Juice of ¼ lemon

2 teaspoon ground turmeric

120g skinless, boneless chicken breast

For the salsa

Juice of ¼ lemon

5g finely chopped parsley

1 tablespoon finely chopped capers

130g tomato (about 1 tomato)

Directions

1. To prepare the salsa, cut off the eye from the tomato and then chop the tomato finely while being careful to retain as much juice as possible.

2. Put the tomato and juice with lemon juice, parsley, and capers in a blender and process.

3. Preheat your oven to 220 degrees Celsius. Meanwhile, marinate the chicken in a teaspoon of little oil, lemon juice, and turmeric.

4. Let the chicken marinate for approximately 5 to 10 minutes. Meanwhile, heat an ovenproof pan until very hot and then add in the marinated chicken.

5. Cook the chicken until pale golden or for about 1 minute on each side. Transfer the frying pan to the oven. In case the pan isn't ovenproof, transfer the chicken to a baking sheet instead.

6. Bake the chicken until it's cooked through, or for approximately 8 to 10 minutes and then remove from the oven.

7. Cover the cooked chicken with foil and let it lest for about 5 more minutes and then serve.

8. As the chicken cools down, place the kale in a steamer and cook for around 5 minutes or so.

9. Fry the ginger and red onions in a little oil until soft and then add in the steamed kale. Fry the contents for 1 more minute.

10. Now cook the buckwheat as per the package directions along with the reserved teaspoon of turmeric.

11. Serve the buckwheat with the veggies, salsa, and the chicken.

Stir-Fry with Noodles

Serves 1

Ingredients

5g celery leaves

100ml chicken stock

50g kale, roughly chopped

75g green beans, chopped

40g celery, trimmed and sliced

20g red onions, sliced

1 teaspoon fresh ginger, finely chopped

1 garlic clove, finely chopped

75g buckwheat noodles

2 teaspoon extra virgin olive oil

2 teaspoon tamari or soy sauce

150g shelled raw king prawns, deveined

Directions

1. Heat a frying pan over high heat. Once hot enough, cook the prawns in a teaspoon of oil and a teaspoon of tamari for approximately 2 to 3 minutes.

2. Transfer the prawns to a plate and then wipe the pan clean using a kitchen paper and set aside.

3. Cook the noodles in boiling water as per the package directions or for approximately 5 to 8 minutes. Drain the noodles and set aside.

4. Fry the red onion, chili, garlic, kale, beans, and celery in the reserved oil for 2 to 3 minutes over medium-high heat.

5. Add in the chicken stock and bring the mixture to a boil, and then simmer until the veggies are well cooked but crunchy, or for 1 to 2 minutes.

6. Add in the celery leaves, noodles, and the prawns to the pan and bring the mixture to a boil.

7. Finally, remove from the heat and enjoy.

Buckwheat Tabouleh

Serves 1

Ingredients

30g rocket or arugula

Juice of ½ lemon

1 tablespoons extra virgin olive oil

100g strawberries, hulled

30g parsley

1 tablespoons capers

25g Medjool dates, pitted

20g red onion

65g tomato

80g avocado

1 tablespoons ground turmeric

50g buckwheat

Directions

1. First, cook the buckwheat along with turmeric as per the package directions.

2. Then drain the buckwheat and let it cool down for a few minutes.

3. Meanwhile chop the parsley, capers, dates, red onion, tomato and avocado and mix the ingredients with the buckwheat.

4. Slice the strawberries and slowly incorporate them into the salad along with lemon juice and oil.

5. Serve the buckwheat tabouleh on a bed of arugula if you like.

Buckwheat Pasta with Broccoli

Serves 3-4

Ingredients

1 teaspoon vegetable broth, yeast free

1 teaspoon oregano

1 tablespoon lemon juice, fresh

3 carrots, sliced

3 tomatoes, diced

1 big broccoli head, florets

1 red bell pepper, sliced into strips

1 white onion, cut in half rings

2 garlic cloves, diced

500g buckwheat pasta

4 tablespoons extra virgin olive oil

Sea salt

Fresh pepper

Directions

1. Cut all the veggies you want to cook and then heat some water seasoned with salt.

2. Cook the broccoli and the buckwheat pasta but in two separate pots.

3. As they cook, add 2 tablespoons of olive oil in a pan and heat it on medium heat.

4. Sauté garlic and onions until translucent, as you stir regularly. Once done, remove from heat and set it aside.

5. In the same pan, add 2 tablespoons of olive oil and cook the veggies until firm to bite. Start with carrots, the bell peppers, and at the end, add in the tomatoes.

6. Drain and add in the broccoli and onions to the pan and season the mixture with vegetable broth, oregano, lemon juice, salt, and pepper.

7. Distribute the veggie-mix over the buckwheat pasta.

8. You can top with some fresh basil if you like.

Chili Chicken Thighs

Serves 4

Ingredients

1 tablespoon chili powder

2 pounds boneless chicken thighs

Lime wedges for serving

Fresh cilantro for garnish

Directions

1. Preheat the oven to 375 degrees F. Drizzle olive oil on the chicken and turn it around to coat.

2. Season with salt, chili powder, and pepper and roast the chicken for 15 minutes.

3. Remove from the oven once the time lapses and sprinkle with cilantro. Serve mushrooms (recipe below) garnished with lime wedges.

Sirtfood Mushrooms

Serves 6

Ingredients

3 cloves garlic, minced

½ lemon

1 ½ teaspoon coarse salt

3 tablespoons olive oil, extra-virgin

2 tablespoons flat-leaf parsley, chopped

1/4 teaspoon black pepper, freshly ground

1 ½ pounds mushroom, fresh

Directions

1. Submerge the mushrooms in water and swish them to clean thoroughly, and drain completely. Trim and slice your mushrooms to bite-sizes.

2. Place the mushrooms in a bowl and squeeze the juice from the lemon half into them. Toss the ingredients completely.

3. In a large pan, add garlic and then pour olive oil. Heat the mixture over medium-high heat until the garlic begins to sizzle. Heat for just 30 seconds to ensure the contents do not brown.

4. Now add in the mushrooms, stir, and cover. Continue cooking while stirring occasionally; say at intervals of around 4 minutes.

5. Once cooked through, remove the lid and add the salt and pepper, and continue cooking. After about 5 minutes, your mushrooms should begin to brown, and all moisture should have evaporated.

6. Now stir in the parsley and then serve.

Coconut Chicken

Serves: 4

Ingredients

8 oz. coconut milk canned

1/4 cup water

1/2 teaspoon Sea Salt

1/2 teaspoon black pepper

1 lb. boneless skinless, chicken thighs

4 tablespoons apple cider vinegar

5 cloves garlic roughly crushed and skins removed

1 tablespoon coconut oil

Directions

1. Add coconut oil and the diced chicken to a medium saucepan. Cook over medium or low heat for about 2 or 3 minutes.

2. Add in garlic cloves, apple cider vinegar, and water and cook for around 3 minutes.

3. Season with salt and pepper and cook for about 10 minutes, or until all the liquids boil down.

4. Add in coconut milk and simmer the mixture until the liquid slightly thickens to form gravy, or for around 5 minutes.

5. Remove from heat, and serve. Do not leave the pan on the heat, as the gravy will cook away, leaving behind coconut oil.

Baked Meatballs

Serves 3

Ingredients

1/4 cup fresh rosemary, roughly chopped

2 garlic cloves, minced

1/2 medium yellow onion, minced

1 teaspoon salt

1/2 teaspoon pepper

1 tablespoon apple cider vinegar

2 tablespoons grass-fed ghee

1 1/4 pounds pastured ground beef

Optional:

1 teaspoon crushed red pepper flakes

Directions

1. Preheat your oven to 350 degrees F. Meanwhile, add all ingredients into a mixing bowl and mix using your hands.

2. Once well-mixed set aside. Line your baking tray with parchment papers.

3. Roll the mixture into small balls, with about 1 tablespoon of mixture per each meatball.

4. As soon as you're done rolling, put them on the parchment-lined baking tray. Bake until cooked through, or for approximately 20 minutes.

5. Serve the meatballs warm, or instead store them in a sealed airtight container in the freezer or refrigerator.

6. You can also meal prep the meatballs, by first letting them cool, then seal in an airtight container. Keep it frozen until ready to cook.

7. To cook, just thaw in the fridge and then reheat in your oven, or add them to a hot sauce.

Lentil Soup

Serves 6

Ingredients

Kosher salt and black pepper

1 tablespoon fresh thyme

½ cup brown lentils

1 bunch kale leaves cut into 1/2-inch-wide strips

2 sweet potatoes, peeled and cut into 1/2-inch pieces

1 28-ounce can whole tomatoes, drained

4 leeks cut into 1/4-inch-thick half-moons

1 tablespoon olive oil

Directions

1. In a Dutch oven or large saucepan, heat some oil over medium heat and then add in the leeks. Cook the onion for approximately 3-4 minutes or until well softened, while stirring now and again.

2. Add in tomatoes and cook for around 5 minutes, while you break them with a spoon.

3. Add in about 6 cups of water to the cooking pan and then bring it to a boil. Stir in ¼ teaspoon pepper, 1 ½ teaspoons salt, thyme, lentils, kales, and sweet potatoes.

4. Simmer the mixture for around 25-30 minutes or until the lentils become tender.

5. You can then spoon the dish into bowls and serve.

Tandoori Tofu

Serves: 6

Ingredients

6 tablespoons sliced cilantro or scallions

2/3 cup plain yogurt, non-fat

2 14-ounce packages tofu, water-packed and drained

1 tablespoon lime juice

1 tablespoon garlic, minced

3 tablespoons olive oil

1/4 teaspoon turmeric, ground

1/2 teaspoon coriander, ground

1/2 teaspoon cumin, ground

1 teaspoon salt, divided

2 teaspoons paprika

Directions

1. Heat your grill to medium-high heat. Meanwhile, start preparing the other ingredients.

2. In a small bowl, mix paprika, turmeric, coriander, cumin, and ½ teaspoon salt to make a spice mixture.

3. In a skillet, heat some oil over medium heat and add in the spice mixture, lime juice, and garlic and stir.

4. Cook for about a minute or until it's sizzling and fragrant, and then remove from heat.

5. Cut the tofu block crosswise into six equal slices and pat dry them. Brush both sides of the sliced tofu with approximately three tablespoons of spiced oil.

6. Also, sprinkle the tofu with ½ teaspoon of salt. Reserve some of the excess spiced oil.

7. Oil the grill rack, and then grill the tofu for 2-3 minutes, or until the grill marks are heated through.

8. In a small bowl, mix the reserved spiced oil with yogurt.

9. You can serve the dish with yogurt sauce while garnished with cilantro or scallions if you like.

Dinner Recipes

Grilled Lamb Chops

Serves 4

Ingredients

8 4-ounce lamb loin chops, trimmed

1/2 teaspoon black pepper, freshly ground

3/4 teaspoon kosher salt, divided

2 garlic cloves, minced

1/8 teaspoon red pepper, crushed

2 teaspoons shallots, minced

1 1/2 tablespoons white vinegar

2 tablespoons lower-sodium chicken broth, fat-free

2 1/2 tablespoons extra-virgin olive oil

1/2 cup fresh flat-leaf parsley

1 1/2 cups fresh mint

Cooking spray

Directions

1. In a food processor, mix ¼ teaspoon pepper, ¼ teaspoon salt, red pepper, shallots, vinegar, broth, oil, parsley, oil, and mint. Process until the ingredients are fully incorporated.

2. Sprinkle lamb loin chops with the remaining salt and pepper on both sides.

3. Heat a grill pan over medium heat. Using some cooking spray, coat a cooking pan well.

4. Put the seasoned lamb onto the spray-coated pan and cook both sides each for approximately for 5 minutes.

5. Once done, serve, and enjoy.

Garlic Chicken

Serves: 4-6

Ingredients

¼ teaspoon pepper

1 1/2 teaspoon crushed basil

1 1/2 lbs cherry tomatoes

2 lbs. chicken cutlets

1 tablespoon chopped garlic- about 4 cloves

¾ cup diced red onion

½ teaspoon salt

2 tablespoon olive oil

Directions

1. Over medium heat, heat oil in a large skillet, and then add in onion and garlic. Cook for about 5 minutes. You should regularly mix the ingredients using a spatula.

2. Add the chicken into the pan and cook for about 3-4 minutes on each side until browned. Thicker chicken breasts may take longer, about 6-8 minutes.

3. Chop the cherry tomatoes in a blender or food processor. Add to the pan with the chicken and stir.

4. Add in pepper, salt, and basil and heat until the boiling. Allow to simmer for about 25 minutes before serving.

Riced Cauliflower With Shrimp

Serves 4

Ingredients

2 teaspoons extra-virgin olive oil

Juice from half a lime

1 teaspoon smoked paprika

1 teaspoon cumin

2 teaspoons curry powder

3/4 cup low-sodium chicken stock

2 tablespoons parsley chopped

1 lb. uncooked shrimp peeled and deveined

2 cloves garlic minced

1/2 red pepper chopped

1 onion chopped

1 bag green giant riced cauliflower frozen

Salt + pepper to taste

Directions

1. In a skillet, over medium heat, add some olive oil.

2. Once hot, add in chopped red pepper and onions and then season with pepper and salt.

3. Cook until soft, or for approximately 3 or 4 minutes.

4. Add in the garlic and cook for another 1 minute or so.

5. Add all the riced cauliflower into the skillet and blend the mixture using a wooden spoon.

6. Add in smoked paprika, curry, and cumin and stir to mix.

7. Add in the chicken broth and reduce the heat to medium-low.

8. Season the uncooked shrimp with salt and pepper and then nestle them over the riced cauliflower.

9. Cook until the shrimp is just cooked through, or for approximately 2 to 3 minutes.

10. Uncover the shrimp and add in some parsley. Squeeze in some lime juice and stir.

11. Taste and adjust the seasoning as required and then remove from heat and serve.

Beef Stir Fry

Serves 4

Ingredients

3-inch scallion green part

3-inch scallion white part

2 red chili peppers thinly sliced

Ginger 3″ long thin slices

3 tablespoons garlic, minced

2 tablespoons toasted sesame oil

1 tablespoon fish sauce

2 tablespoons coconut aminos

Olive oil

1 lb. beef tips thinly sliced

Directions

1. In a bowl, whisk together sesame oil, fish sauce, and coconut aminos. Drizzle this on the beef tips and marinate the meat for approximately 15 to 30 minutes.

2. Drizzle some oil in a large skillet and cook the beef tips for about 3 minutes, or until no longer pink.

3. Remove the beef from the skillet and set it aside.

4. Add in white scallion pieces, garlic, chili peppers, and ginger in the same pan.

5. Add in green scallion pieces and beef and toss until well combined. Serve and enjoy.

Turkey Breast Tenderloin

Serves 2

Ingredients

1/4 teaspoon pepper

1 teaspoon salt

1/4 teaspoon sage

1/4 teaspoon thyme

1/2 teaspoon rosemary

1 teaspoon garlic powder

2 turkey breast tenderloin about 24 ounces

1 cup broth or water

Directions

1. Rub the spices and the herbs onto the meat and then put the turkey into the instant pot.

2. Lock the lid in place and press on the "Poultry" setting and adjust cooking time to 7 to 10 minutes depending on the size of the turkey fillets.

3. As soon as the turkey is ready, quick release the pressure and open the lid. Remove the cooked turkey breast.

4. You can serve the liquid from the cooking pan with meat or save it as broth for another recipe.

Lamb And Ginger Stir Fry

Serves 4

Ingredients

9 oz lamb, minced

1 tablespoon sunflower oil

1 tablespoon, chopped or grated fresh root ginger

1 medium onion, chopped

1 medium green pepper, chopped

1 medium red pepper, chopped

1 teaspoon black pepper, ground to taste

Directions

1. Fry the minced lamb meat in sunflower oil at a high temperature until browned, or for about 3 to 4 minutes.

2. Add in the peppers, onion and root ginger and fry for another 2 to 3 minutes, while stirring continuously.

3. Season the dish with some pepper and then serve.

Kale Salad

Serves 2-3

Ingredients

1/2 red onion, very thinly sliced

2 bunches kale

6 Medjool dates, pitted

1/3 cup whole hazelnuts

For the dressing

5 tablespoons toasted hazelnut oil

Pinch of coarse salt

1 Medjool date

4 tablespoons orange juice, freshly squeezed

2 tablespoons raw apple cider vinegar

Directions

1. Preheat the oven to 375 degrees F and then put the hazelnuts onto a baking dish. Roast the nuts for about 7-8 minutes, or until the skin begins to darken and split.

2. Once done, transfer the nuts while still hot and let them steam for 15 minutes while wrapped in a kitchen towel.

3. Once cooled down, squeeze and twist around firmly to remove the skin, all this time still wrapped in the towel.

4. Into a food processor, put the pitted dates along with the hazelnuts and pulse them until finely chopped. Set it aside to top the salad.

5. Wash, dry and chop the kale and then put it in a large bowl. Slice the onion thinly and add it into the bowl.

6. Prepare the dressing by combining the ingredients for "dressing" in the blender apart from the hazelnut oil.

7. Puree the mixture to break down the dates and then drizzle the oil in a steady stream to emulsify the dressing.

8. Finally, toss the kale and onion mixture along with the orange-hazelnut dressing.

9. Transfer to a platter bowl and sprinkle with the hazelnut and dates mixture. Enjoy!

Zucchini Pasta

Serves 4

Ingredients

Olive oil

2 cloves garlic

4 tomatoes

12 basil leaves

1 bunch asparagus

1/2 red onion

1 bag of rocket

1 zucchini

Directions

1. Make noodle-shaped strips from the zucchini using a spiralizer. Put this in boiling water for a few minutes, remove from heat and drain. Drizzle with some oil in case the strips look sticky.

2. Meanwhile, chop the tomatoes into chunks and dice the onion. Place them on one side with a couple of rocket.

3. Start making the sauce. Mix the asparagus, the rocket leaves, 1 cup of chopped zucchini, garlic and basil in a blender and process.

4. As you blend, drizzle olive oil until you get a sauce that is thick and light green in color. Season the sauce with salt and pepper.

5. Stir the sauce with the zucchini noodles and put into serving bowls. Top with arugula, red onion and tomato.

Chicken Piccata

Serves 4

Ingredients

5 ounces Baby portabella mushrooms, sliced

1/3 cup fresh parsley chopped

1/4 cup capers

1/2 cup low-sodium chicken broth

1/3 cup fresh lemon juice

6 tablespoons coconut oil

5 tablespoons extra-virgin olive oil

1/3 cup almond flour

2 boneless chicken breasts, butter fried

Pepper to taste

Salt to taste

Directions

1. Generously season the chicken with salt and pepper. Pour the almond flour into a large bowl and dredge both sides of the seasoned chicken in the flour. Shake off any excess almond flour from the meat.

2. Heat 3 tablespoons of olive oil along with 2 tablespoons of coconut oil in a large skillet over medium high heat.

3. Add the two pieces of chicken as soon as the oil mixture begins to sizzle and cook the meat until browned, or for approximately 3 minutes on each side.

4. Flip and cook the other side too. Once done, transfer the cooked chicken to a serving plate.

5. Heat 2 tablespoons of olive oil along with 2 tablespoons of coconut oil in a skillet until the mixture begins to sizzle.

6. Add the second batch of 2 pieces of chicken to the hot oil and brown both sides say for about 3 minutes per side.

7. Add in the mushrooms into the pan and cook for approximately 5 minutes. Remove the hot pan from heat and transfer the chicken to a plate.

8. Add chicken broth, capers and lemon juice to the pan. Set on a stove and bring the mixture to a boil. Keep scraping any browned bits from the pan to enhance flavor.

9. Taste and adjust the seasoning as required, then return the cooked chicken to the pan.

10. Simmer for around 5 minutes or so then move the meat to a serving dish. Add in the reserved 2 tablespoons of coconut oil to the sauce and whisk to incorporate.

11. Pour the sauce over the meat and serve garnished with parsley.

Snacks and Appetizers

Dark Chocolate Bites

Serves 15-20 bites

Ingredients

1–2 tablespoons water

1 teaspoon vanilla extract or scraped seeds of 1 vanilla pod

1 tablespoon extra virgin olive oil

1 tablespoon ground turmeric

1 tablespoon cocoa powder

250g Medjool dates, pitted

30g dark chocolate or cocoa nibs

120g walnuts

Directions

1. Put the chocolate and the walnuts in a food processor and blend until you have a fine powder.

2. Add the rest of the ingredients apart from the water and process until you get a ball.

3. You can add in water if necessary depending on the consistency of the dough to avoid it from becoming too sticky.

4. Form the dough into bite-sized balls using your hands and keep them refrigerated in an airtight container for a minimum of 1 hour.

5. You can roll a few of the balls in desiccated coconut or cocoa if you like. The bites can be refrigerated up to 7 days.

Chocolate Raspberry Cups

Serves 1

Ingredients

4 tablespoons coconut, shredded

1/2 tablespoon stevia powder + 1 teaspoon

1/2 cup raspberries

1 tablespoon water

5 tablespoons raw cocoa powder + 1 tablespoon

Directions

1. To make the filling, mix cocoa powder, stevia, water and raspberries in a blender and process until smooth.

2. To make the cups, use silicon cup moulds. Mix a tablespoon of coconut water, stevia and shredded coconut in a bowl.

3. Add in some water and mix it together using your hands. Line the inside of the cupcake moulds with the shredded coconut paste.

4. Fill the cupcakes with the raspberry chocolate filling and keep chilled for a couple of hours to harden and solidify.

5. Once very solid, remove from the fridge and serve.

Sweet Potato Chips

Serves 10

Ingredients

Pepper to taste

2 sweet potatoes

2 tablespoons coconut oil

1 teaspoon pure sea salt

Directions

1. Preheat your oven to 375 degrees F.

2. Using a sharp knife, slice your sweet potatoes to bite-sizes and then toss together with coconut oil, salt, pepper and rosemary to season. Ensure you rub the sweet potatoes fully in oil to coat.

3. Using a parchment paper, line your baking sheet and then arrange your sweet potatoes on it.

4. Bake the contents in the preheated oven for 25-30 minutes. To ensure they bake well with a crispier texture, flip the potatoes once.

5. Once crispy brown with soft centers, remove from heat and let them cool to harden.

Yogurt Pops

Serves 8

Ingredients

8 – 10 drops liquid stevia

4 tablespoons lemon juice, divided

2 cups Greek yogurt, divided

1/2 cup blueberries, chopped

1/2 cup strawberries, chopped

Directions

1. Mix half the yogurt, straw berries, the sweetener and a tablespoon of lemon juice in a food processor or blender.

2. Puree until smooth and then transfer to a measuring cup or a bowl. Add into the blender, a tablespoon of lemon juice, half-cup yogurt, preferred sweetener and blueberries.

3. Puree until the contents have blended well.

4. Distribute the strawberry mixture among 8 paper cups or popsicle molds. Firmly tap the molds on the counter to make it settle.

5. Distribute the yogurt mixture among cups or molds and tap firmly. Top the contents with the blueberry mixture and tap it well too.

6. Put the molds in a freezer and keep frozen for about 1 hour. As soon as they begin to firm up, add in the popsicle sticks and freeze for another 2 to 3 hours, or until firm.

7. In case you want to go red, white and red, it's recommended to use 1 cup of strawberries while omitting the blueberries.

8. Just process the strawberries with 2 tablespoons of lemon juice, a cup of yogurt and a sweetener of your choice.

9. Then layer the mixture on the bottom and at the top of your molds.

Crispy Zucchini Fries

Serves 4

Ingredients

1/4 teaspoon garlic powder

1 large egg

3/4 cup grated Parmesan cheese

2 medium zucchini

1/4 teaspoon black pepper, optional

Directions

1. Preheat your oven to 425 degrees F and then line your baking sheet with foil or parchment paper. Lightly grease the baking sheet.

2. Cut individual zucchini in half lengthwise a couple of times until you have 8 long sticks from each of the squash.

3. Cut the 8 sticks crosswise to have a total of 16 sticks that measure about 10 centimeters or 4 inches long. In case the zucchini sticks appear wet just pat them dry with a paper towel.

4. Set up two shallow bowls, one with the grated cheese, black pepper and garlic mixture and the other with 1 beaten egg.

5. Dip individual sticks into the egg, shake off any excess egg and press into the Parmesan and garlic mixture to coat all the sides. You can use one of your hands in the egg and the other for the cheese mixture.

6. Put the squash on the lined baking sheet in a single layer, ensuring they do not touch.

7. Bake in the preheated oven for approximately 20 minutes, while rotating the pan and flipping the fries while halfway through, until the zucchini is fairly dark golden.

8. Put the dish under the broiler and broil until dark golden and crispy, or for approximately 2 to 3 minutes.

Sirtfood Garlic Mushrooms

Serves: 2-3

Ingredients

A pinch of black pepper

2 pinches of sea salt

1 1/2 tablespoon ghee

Zest of 1 lemon + a drizzle of lemon juice

1 garlic clove, peeled and diced

5 springs of fresh thyme, leaves only

4 cups sliced button mushrooms

Directions

1. In a large frying pan, heat some ghee until hot and then add in thyme and mushrooms.

2. Cook the mixture on high until browned, and then lower the heat to medium.

3. Add in garlic, pepper, lemon zest and sea salt and cook for about 5-6 minutes. Stir a few times.

1. Add in more fresh thyme and a drizzle of fresh lemon juice. If you like it, add some splash of truffle oil and then serve.

Salmon Salad

Serves 1

Ingredients

10g celery leaves, chopped

10g parsley, chopped

Juice of ¼ lemon

1 tablespoon extra-virgin olive oil

1 large Medjool date, pitted and chopped

1 tablespoon capers

15g walnuts, chopped

20g red onion, sliced

40g celery, sliced

80g avocado, peeled, stoned and sliced

100g smoked salmon slices,

50g chicory leaves

50g rocket

Directions

1. Layer the salad leaves on a bowl or a large plate.

2. Combine the rest of the ingredients together and serve the salad on top of the salad leaves.

Sirtfood Salad

Serves 1

Ingredients

¼ cup parsley, chopped

Juice of ¼ lemon

1 tablespoon extra virgin olive oil

1 large Medjool date, pitted and chopped

1 tablespoon capers

⅛ cups walnuts, chopped

⅛ cup red onion, sliced

½ cup celery including leaves, sliced

½ cup avocado, peeled, stoned, and sliced

3 ½ ounces smoked salmon slices

1 ¾ ounces endive leaves

1 ¾ ounces arugula

Directions

1. Put the salad leaves in a large bowl or on a plate.

2. Combine the rest of the ingredients together and serve on the salad leaves.

Hearty Lentil Salad

Serves 2

Ingredients

1 cup canned or cooked lentils

2 cups arugula

Kosher salt

Pepper

2 cloves garlic, mashed

2 sprigs thyme

1/2 teaspoon cumin

1 tablespoon olive oil

1 apple, cut into medium dices

2 cups peeled butternut squash

Directions

1. Preheat your oven to 375 degrees F. Line a parchment paper on baking sheet and toss apple and squash with oil, garlic, thyme and cumin.

2. Season with salt, pepper, and roast for about 20 minutes or until the squash is tender. Allow to cool for some time.

3. Divide the lentils, apple, squash, and arugula between two plates and drizzle with olive oil. Season the dish with pepper and salt.

Sirtfood Greek Salad

Serves 8

Ingredients

1/2 red onion, sliced

1/3 cup sun-dried tomatoes, diced

3 cups roma tomatoes, diced

1 cup black olives, pitted and sliced

1 1/2 cups crumbled feta cheese

3 cucumbers, seeded and sliced

Directions

1. Toss together sun-dried tomatoes, roma tomatoes, olives, feta cheese, cucumbers, tomato oil and red onion in a large bowl.

2. Keep the mixture chilled until you are ready to serve.

Green Juices

Sirtfood Green Juice

Serves 1

Ingredients

1/2 teaspoon matcha green tea

1/2 lemon

1/2 green apple

1 cm ginger piece

2 celery sticks

5 grams parsley

1 oz. arugula

2.5 oz. kale

Directions

1. Add all the ingredients to a juicer apart from the lemon and green tea.

2. Juice them and pour the mixture into a glass.

3. Squeeze the juice from the lemon into a cup.

4. Stir in both the green tea powder and the lemon juice in the juice.

Sirtfood Juice

Serves 1

Ingredients

Pinch of black pepper

Juice of ¼ lemon

½ medium apple, unpeeled

4–6 cm fresh ginger, peeled

3–5 cm turmeric root, peeled

Directions

1. First, juice the apple, ginger and turmeric.

2. Squeeze in lemon juice or instead peel the lemon and add it to the juicer as whole.

3. Now grind some black pepper and stir the juice.

Collard Juice

Serves 2

Ingredients

1/2 medium lime, peeled

1/2 medium lemon, peeled

2 stalks celery

1/2 medium cucumber

2 1/2 medium apples

2 leaves collard greens

Directions

1. In a juicer, mix medium-sized lime, medium-lemon, stalks celery, cucumber, and apples.

2. If you do not have a juicer, you can also process the ingredients in a blender and then add water to make juice.

Beet Root Juice

Serves 32 oz

Ingredients

2 oranges (peeled)

½ lemon

12 carrots

1 beet root - (3 inches diameter)

1 apple

Directions

1. Into your juicer, combine oranges, lemon, carrots, beetroot and medium apple and process until ready.

2. Stir, and then serve and enjoy!

Grapefruit Mint Juice

Serves 1

Ingredients

1 lemon

2 grapefruits

5 sprigs fresh mint

5 sprigs fresh basil

2 cucumbers

Directions

1. Wash all the ingredients, peel the grape fruit and lemon and then separate the mint and basil leaves from the stems; get rid of the stems.

2. Add basil and mint leaves along with peeled lemon and grapefruit to a juicer.

3. Process then serve.

Sirtfood Juice

Serves 2 glasses

Ingredients

1/2 medium lemon, peeled

1 inch fresh ginger-root, peeled

1/2 medium cucumber

1 cup spinach

1 cup kale

2 leaves collard greens

2 leaves Swiss chard

Directions

1. Mix together lemon, ginger-root, cucumber, spinach, kale, collard greens and Swiss chard in a juicer and process.

2. Enjoy!

Cucumber Parsley Juice

Serves: 1

Ingredients

2 cups baby spinach

1 lemon, peeled

1 cup fresh parsley

¼ cup fresh mint

1 medium pear

1 large cucumber

Directions

1.   Process all the above ingredients in a blender or juicer.

2.   Pour into a glass and then serve.

Cilantro Apple Juice

Serves: 1

Ingredients

½ lemon, peeled

¼ cup fresh cilantro

1 medium cucumber

2 large kale leaves

2 stalks celery

2 green apples

Directions

1. Process all the ingredients in your juicer.

2. Stir the juice then serve and enjoy.

Sirtfood Go-To Drink

Serves 2

Ingredients

1/2 medium lemon, peeled

1 sprig fresh mint

2 medium green apples

1/2 cup pineapple

1/2 small beet

1/2 cup parsley

2 leaves Swiss chard

1 cup kale

Directions

1. To make the juice, put all the ingredients in your juicer.

2. Process and then pour into a cup. Serve.

Healthy Homemade Juice

Serves 1

Ingredients

4-10 mint leaves (for flavor)

6 strawberries

Handful of blueberries

2 kiwis

2 apples

Directions

1. Add all ingredients into a juicer or blender.

2. Puree and then serve.

Green Tea Smoothie

Serves 2

Ingredients

2 teaspoons honey

6 ice cubes

1/2 teaspoon vanilla bean paste or a seeds from a vanilla pod

2 teaspoons matcha green tea powder

250 ml almond milk

2 ripe bananas

Directions

1. Add all the ingredients in a blender and blend until smooth.

2. Serve and enjoy.

Tonic Green Smoothie

Serves 1

Ingredients

1 cup of water

Juice of 1/2 lime

Juice of 1/2 lemon

3 Granny Smith apples

2 celery sticks

1/2 medium size cucumber

1 handful of parsley

1 cup of kale

Directions

1. Add water to a high-powered blender along with parsley and kale. Process the ingredients until smooth.

2. Add cucumber, and celery and process again.

3. Add lemon and lime juices and the apples and puree until smooth.

4. Enjoy!

Green Smoothie

Serves 1

Ingredients

1 handful of ice

1 cup of cold water

1 lemon wedge, peeled

2 cups of fresh baby spinach or kale

1/2 cup of green grapes

1/2 kiwi, peeled

Directions

1. First, peel the lemon and discard the seeds. Also peel the kiwi.

2. Put the lemon along with the half a kiwi in a blender.

3. Add the rest of the contents in the blender and process until smooth.

4. Serve immediately.

Ultimate Green Smoothie

Serves 1

Ingredients

Juice from ½ lemon

2 cups spinach, tightly packed

1 apple, cored

1 frozen banana, optional

1 cup strawberries, frozen

1 cup water

½ cup chopped cucumber

Ice, optional

Directions

1. In a blender, combine 2 cups of freshly packed spinach with the apple, juice from half lemon, frozen strawberries and a cup of water.

2. If you like, incorporate a frozen banana or additional ice.

3. Process the ingredients for a few seconds until ready.

4. To lower the sugar or level of calories, omit one fruit serving and then add in stevia sweetener.

5. You can also add in a tablespoon of milled flax seeds or chia seeds to get extra healthy fats.

Sweet Spinach Smoothie

Serves 2

Ingredients

1 or 2 tablespoons fresh lime juice

2 tablespoons chopped avocado

6 ounces fat-free plain Greek yogurt

15 green or red grapes

1 ripe pear, peeled, cored, and chopped

2 cups spinach leaves, packed

Directions

1. Add all the ingredients into your blender.

2. Puree until smooth or preferred consistency.

Green Tea Smoothie

Serves 1

Ingredients

1/2 banana

1 tablespoon raw honey

1 teaspoon cinnamon

1/2 cup almond milk, unsweetened

1/2 cup green tea, chilled

Directions

1. In a blender, add 1-2 scoops of ice together with the other ingredients. Process until done.

2. Serve instantly or reserve the tea in the fridge until ready to use. If you like, consider adding other ingredients like spinach or kale for more detox benefits.

Blueberry and Banana smoothie

Serves: 1

Ingredients

¾ cup vanilla soy milk, calcium fortified

½ medium banana

1½ cup frozen blueberries

2 teaspoons honey

1 green tea bag

3 tablespoons water

Directions

1. In a small bowl, microwave the water on high until it starts to steam.

2. Add in the tea bag and let it to brew for about 3 minutes, and then take out the tea bag.

3. Stir honey into the tea and stir thoroughly to allow it to dissolve.

4. Add milk, banana and berries into a blender that can crush ice and add in the tea.

5. Process the mixture on ice-crush or other higher settings to smoothness. You may need to add in some water in order to process the mixture.

6. Pour the smoothie into a tall glass and serve immediately.

Berry Smoothie

Serves 1

Ingredients

1 tablespoon chia

4 tablespoon almond butter, raw

1 banana, peeled and frozen

1 cup of frozen mixed berries

2 cups almond milk, unsweetened

2 cups fresh spinach

Directions

1. Blend the spinach and almond milk first.

2. Add in the other ingredients apart from chia and blend.

3. Once smooth, add in chia and continue to blend to incorporate.

4. Allow to sit for a few minutes before serving.

Matcha Green Tea Smoothie

Serves: 1-2

Ingredients

1 teaspoon matcha green tea powder

¾ to 1 cup almond milk, unsweetened

5 ice cubes

1 Banana

Directions

1. Into a blender, place the ice cubes and the banana

2. Add in the almond milk followed by the matcha green tea powder.

3. Process the ingredients to achieve a smooth consistency.

4. Pour into a glass and enjoy.

Green Smoothie Bowl

Serves: 2

Ingredients

1 tablespoon almond flakes

1 tablespoon unsweetened coconut

1 teaspoon chia seeds

1 lime, juice only

1 small bunch fresh parsley

1 cup fresh spinach leaves

1 small cucumber, cut in cubes

1 cup coconut water

1 ripe avocado, peeled and cut in cubes

Directions

1. Puree all the ingredients in a blender until you get a creamy smooth mixture.

2. Pour this into a bowl, and top with almonds, coconut and chia seeds if you like.

3. Serve immediately to benefits from benefits offered by these ingredients.

Getting Started on the Sirtfood Diet

The easiest way to succeed in any new diet is to start making small positive changes towards your new dieting lifestyle. Taking off one thing at a time is more effective as opposed to removing everything on the menu that are non-sirtfoods. This way, your brain can adjust. Here are a few steps that can help you get started:

Stock Up Your Kitchen

It takes effort and time to transform your pantry to what sirtfood dieting lifestyle calls for. While it is time consuming, having a variety of foods is important when transiting, as this ensures you get variety of tastes.

Ensure that you have an adequate supply of sirtfood friendly whole foods, fruits and veggies; and then gradually increase the collection of these foods.

Begin to Plan Your Meals

Failing to plan is planning to fail. As you get started, it is advisable to plan your meals so that you can incorporate sirtfoods into your diet and know when you are supposed to eat what. This will avoid instances of eating foods that are not recommended in the sirtfood diet because you just do not have sirtfood friendly foods to eat.

Remember the following rules:

Phase 1

First 3 days of the week

- 3 green juices/smoothie in a day

- 1 sirtfoods meal

Next 4 days

- 2 green juices/smoothie in a day

- 2 main meals

Phase 2

- Goes for 14 days

- Drink just one green juice/smoothie a day

- 3 "balanced" sirtfoods meals

Here is a sample Sirtfood diet meal plan that you can modify as you wish to your dieting needs:

3 Weeks Meal plan

Phase 1

Day 1

Breakfast

Green Tea Smoothie

Lunch

Sirtfood Green Juice

Dinner

Grilled Lamb Chops

Snack

Sirtfood Juice

Day 2

Breakfast

Tonic Green Smoothie

Lunch

Collard Cooler Juice

Dinner

Garlic chicken

Snack

Beetroot juice

Day 3

Breakfast

Green Smoothie

Lunch

Grapefruit Mint Juice

Dinner

Riced Cauliflower with Shrimp

Snack

Sirtfood Juice

Day 4

Breakfast

Ultimate Green Smoothie

Lunch

Chicken thighs

Dinner

Beef Stir Fry

Snack

Cucumber Parsley Juice

Day 5

Breakfast

Sweet Spinach Smoothie

Lunch

Chicken breast with kale

Dinner

Turkey Breast Tenderloin

Snack

Cilantro Apple Green Juice

Day 6

Breakfast

Green Tea Smoothie

Lunch

Prawn stir-fry with buckwheat noodles

Dinner

Chicken Piccata

Snack

Sirtfood Go-To Drink

Day 7

Breakfast

Blueberry, and Banana smoothie

Lunch

Strawberry buckwheat tabouleh

Dinner

Lamb and Ginger Stir Fry

Snack

Healthy Homemade Juice

Phase 2

Week 1

Day 8

Breakfast

Berry Smoothie

Lunch

Buckwheat Pasta with Broccoli

Dinner

Zucchini Sauté

Snack

Dark Chocolate Bites

Day 9

Breakfast

Almond Milk Smoothie

Lunch

Roasted Chicken Thighs

Dinner

Kale Salad

Snack

Chocolate Raspberry Cups

Day 10

Breakfast

Green Smoothie Bowl

Lunch

Roasted Chicken Thighs

Dinner

Zucchini Pasta

Snack

Sweet Potato Chips

Day 11

Breakfast

Sirtfood Green Juice

Lunch

Sirtfood Mushrooms

Dinner

Chicken Piccata

Snack

Sweet Potato Chips

Day 12

Breakfast

Breakfast Scramble

Lunch

Easy Coconut Chicken

Dinner

Grilled Lamb Chops

Snack

Sirtfood Juice

Day 13

Breakfast

Green Tea Smoothie

Lunch

Baked Meatballs

Dinner

Garlic chicken

Snack

Yogurt Pops

Day 14

Breakfast

Matcha Overnight Oats

Lunch

Lentil Soup

Dinner

Riced Cauliflower with Shrimp

Snack

Collard Cooler Juice

Phase 3

Week 2

Day 15

Breakfast

Healthy Homemade Juice

Lunch

Tandoori Tofu

Dinner

Beef Stir Fry

Snack

Zucchini Fries

Day 16

Breakfast

Sirtfood porridge

Lunch

Prawn stir-fry with buckwheat noodles

Dinner

Turkey Breast Tenderloin

Snack

Beetroot juice

Day 17

Breakfast

Smoked salmon omelet

Lunch

Sirtfood Go-To Drink

Dinner

Kale Salad

Snack

Sirtfood Garlic Mushrooms

Day 18

Breakfast

Veggie Omelet

Lunch

Sirtfood Greek salad

Dinner

Lamb and Ginger Stir Fry

Snack

Grapefruit Juice

Day 19

Breakfast

Breakfast Sausage Patties

Lunch

Green Juice

Dinner

Zucchini Pasta

Snack

Sirtfood Super Salad

Day 20

Breakfast

Breakfast Casserole

Lunch

Lentil Salad

Dinner

Chicken Piccata

Snack

Cucumber Parsley Juice

Day 21

Breakfast

Omelet

Lunch

Cilantro Apple Green Juice

Dinner

Chicken breast with kale

Snack

Sirtfood Super Salad

Conclusion

We have come to the end of the book. Thank you for reading and congratulations on reading until the end.

If you found the book valuable, can you recommend it to others? One way to do that is to post a review on Amazon.

Please leave a review for this book on Amazon by visiting the page below:

https://amzn.to/2VMR5qr

Thank you, and good luck!